2022 GLUTEN FREE BUYERS GUIDE

JOSH SCHIEFFER

Table of Contents

How to Read

Example: Breakfast-On-The-Go

2022 Annual Gluten Free Awards

1st Place Winner: Canyon Bakehouse Honey Whole Grain English Muffins

2nd Place Winner: Schär Cinnamon Raisin Bagels

3rd Place Winner: Goodie Girl Cookies® Blueberry Breakfast Biscuits

Runner Up:

Bobo's Banana Peanut Butter Protein Bar

Other Great Products:

Bakery On Main Organic Probiotic Walnut Banana Premium Oatmeal

Glutino English Muffins

Introduction by Josh Schieffer

This happens to be our ninth Gluten Free Buyers Guide and our 13th year hosting the Annual Gluten Free Awards. If you are not familiar with the book, I thought it would be best to explain what the book is and more importantly what it is not.

This book is much more than a list of great gluten free products to buy, we also list some of the best gluten free personalities. Being on a gluten free diet can be isolating in so many ways. With a heavy emphasis on celiac disease, we produce eye opening information gathered from polling our readers. Our goal is to ensure you do not feel so alone.

This book does not contain every single gluten free product available in every market. The gluten free industry has changed dramatically since we started in 2008. Virtually no regional grocery chains had private label gluten free products and now it is the norm with west coast chains like Safeway and east coast chains like Publix. We tend to focus on brands with national distribution and national grocery chains. We do this so you have access to these products regardless of where you live. Oftentimes ordering online can save you money, time and widen your options dramatically.

You will not find every brand or product listed in this book on your local grocery shelves. It's a strange fact to some but often brands have to pay to sit on the shelves of most grocery stores. This is especially true for products that don't get purchased as often, like gluten free products. If you have a favorite product that your store doesn't carry, you can request that they stock it for a trial period. If it sells, more than likely they will keep it without the brand paying for the space. However, if a competing brand buys out the shelf space your product will more than likely disappear. This is the cold hard truth about the industry. Those of us who eat gluten free food to maintain a healthy lifestyle pay the price. Gluten Free food is our medicine for a diagnosis we didn't want or ask for. Please use this guide to help make your gluten free lifestyle the best it can be.

Why do I tell you all of this? Those of us with restricted diets have limited options especially in rural parts of the country. I do not want your diet and the products you eat being dictated by what brands pay to sit on your local shelves. The product placement in your local store is not based on how great the product is and how well it tastes. If you want to have the best gluten free products in your pantry, more than likely you will need to travel to multiple stores and order online.

At the end of the day, I want you to know that there are great gluten free products for you and your family. If you are new to the gluten free diet or just struggling to maintain the diet because of product availability or poor product quality, we published this book for you. Please read "Our Story" so you have a better understanding of why we have hundreds of product pictures and not just a list of a million random gluten free products.

This year we had nearly 2,000 people take part in the voting process. The individual responses are all rolled up in the following pages. We added a few new gluten free award categories and have organized the book in sections for easier navigation.

Our Story

The story behind The Gluten Free Awards that very few people know

I remember it like it was yesterday when my four-year-old son Jacob, now seveteen, was playing in the kiddie pool with other kids that I assumed were his age based on their height. After asking all the surrounding kids what ages they were, I realized Jacob was significantly smaller than kids his own age. This prompted my wife and I to seek a professional opinion. After consulting with our family physician, she confirmed that Jacob had essentially stopped growing for an entire year without us realizing it. He was referred to Jeff Gordon's Children's Hospital in Charlotte North Carolina to discuss possible growth hormone therapy. The doctors there reviewed Jacob's case and requested a few blood tests based on some suspicions they had.

Our cell phone service at our house was terrible so when the doctor finally called with the blood results, my wife and I ran to the front of the driveway to hear the doctor clearly. With a sporadic signal, we heard "Jacob has celiac disease." We looked at each other as tears ran down my wife's face. We huddled closer to the phone and asked, "what is celiac disease?". After getting a brief description mixed with crappy cell service and happy neighbors waving as they drove by, my wife and I embraced and wept. We were told to maintain his normal diet until we could have an endoscopy and biopsy for further confirmation. Once confirmed our next visit was to a registered dietitian for guidance.

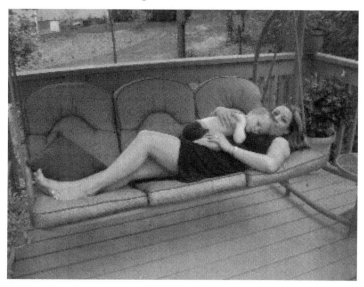

Jayme, my wife, made the appointment and called me with a weird request. "Will you meet me at the dietitian's house for a consultation?". I was confused when she said to go to her house. Jayme then explained that the dietician's daughter had celiac disease too and the best way to show the new lifestyle to patients would be to dive right in. I'll admit, it was a bit uncomfortable at first to be in a strangers' house looking at their personal items but looking back now, I wouldn't change it for the world. That encounter is ultimately the motivation behind The Gluten Free Awards and the associated Gluten Free Buyers Guide. We left her house with complete understanding of cross contamination, best practices and what products they personally liked and disliked. We new what the product packaging looked like and is the reason we have so many product images in the guide.   That visit was life changing and left us feeling confident as we made our way to the local health food store.

That first trip shopping took forever. Each label was read, and cross checked with our list of known gluten containing suspects. It was also shocking to see the bill when it was time to pay. We had replaced our entire pantry and fridge with all products that had the "Gluten Free" label. We both worked full-time and had decent paying jobs and it still set us back financially.

We looked for support groups locally and came across a "100% Gluten-Free Picnic" in Raleigh, which was two hours away from where we lived. This was our first time meeting other people with celiac disease and we were fortunate to have met some informative people that were willing to help with the hundreds of questions we had. We were introduced to a family whose son had been recently diagnosed with celiac disease as well. His condition was much worse than Jacobs and he was almost hospitalized before finally being diagnosed. They confided in us as we shared similar stories. There were two differences that would change my life forever. The first was the fact that they didn't have the same experience with a registered dietitian. Instead, they were handed a two-page Xerox copy of "safe foods". Second, they didn't have the financial security to experiment with gluten free counterparts. Their first two months exposed to the gluten free lifestyle left them extremely depressed and broke.

On our way home from that picnic, Jayme and I felt compelled to help make a difference in some way. We were determined to help that family and others being diagnosed with this disease. Up until that day, we hadn't found a resource that gave unbiased opinions on gluten free products and services. Fast forward a few years and I too was diagnosed with celiac disease. That year, The Gluten Free Awards were born.

Originally our vision was to create a one-page website with a handful of categories organized by peoples' favorites. Since 2010 we have produced The Annual Gluten Free Awards (GFA) growing into over sixty gluten free categories. After several requests, in 2014, we took the GFA results and published our first Gluten Free Buyers Guide. The annual guide is sold primarily in the United States however we continue to see increased global sales. Each year we have people vote for their favorite gluten free products and we now communicate to nearly 25,000 people weekly through our email list.

We want to thank those special people and organizations that brought us to where we are today:

Pat Fogarty MS, RD, LDN for allowing us to enter your home.

Jeff Gordon's Children's Hospital

Raleigh Celiac Support Groups

Dean Meisel, MD, FAAP for the excellent medical care he provides for our family.

I hope you have learned something new from the story behind The Gluten Free Awards. Today, Jacob and I continue to live a healthy gluten free lifestyle.

2022
GFA
Gluten Free Awards
Presented by:
The Gluten Free
Buyers Guide

Bread & Bakery

Bagels

2022 Annual Gluten Free Awards

1st Place Winner: Canyon Bakehouse Everything Bagel

2nd Place Winner: Udi's Whole Grain Bagels

3rd Place Winner: Little Northern Bakehouse Gluten Free Everything Bagels

Runner Up: Trader Joe's Everything Bagel

Other Great Products:

O'Doughs Everything Bagels

Canyon Bakehouse Plain Bagels

So many ways to go
GLUTEN-FREE.

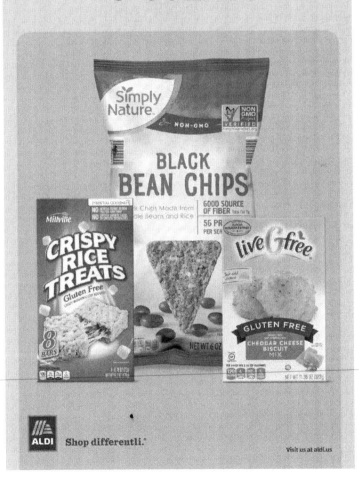

Bread

2022 Annual Gluten Free Awards

1st Place Winner: Canyon Bakehouse Mountain White

2nd Place Winner: Canyon Bakehouse Ancient Grain

3rd Place Winner: Schär Deli Style Sourdough

Runner Up: MYBREAD Gluten Free Bakery Original Baguettes

Other Great Products:

ALDI-exclusive liveGfree White Wide Pan Bread

ALDI-exclusive liveGfree Whole Grain Wide Pan Bread

LIDL Gluten Free Cinnamon Raisin Bread

BFree Panini Rolls

Canyon Bakehouse Hawaiian Sweet

Breadcrumbs

2022 Annual Gluten Free Awards

1st Place Winner: Aleia's Best. Taste. Ever. Italian Bread-crumbs

2nd Place Winner: Aleia's Best. Taste. Ever. Panko

3rd Place Winner: Aleia's Best. Taste. Ever. Coat & Crunch Extra Crispy

Runner Up: 4C Gluten Free Seasoned Breadcrumbs

Other Great Products:

Gillian's Italian GF Breadcrumbs

Ian's Panko Breadcrumbs

Buns

2022 Annual Gluten Free Awards

1st Place Winner: Canyon Bakehouse Stay Fresh Burger Buns

2nd Place Winner: Schär Hamburger Buns

3rd Place Winner: Trader Joe's Gluten Free Hamburger Buns

Runner Up:

Little Northern Bakehouse Millet and Chia Gluten Free Hamburger Bun

Other Great Buns:

Udi's Gluten Free Hamburger Buns

CELIAC SURVEY

We polled over 600 people with celiac disease with the intent to make you feel not so alone.

How long have you had Celiac Disease?

Average length: 16 years

9,494 combined years of experience

Presented by The 2022 Gluten Free Buyers Guide

YOU'RE NOT ALONE

Cookies

2022 Annual Gluten Free Awards

1st Place Winner: Schär Chocolate Honeygrams

2nd Place Winner: OREO Gluten Free Chocolate Sandwich
Cookies

3rd Place Winner: Tate's Bake Shop Gluten Free Chocolate
Chip Cookies

Runner Up: ALDI-exclusive Simply Nature Grain Free Chocolate Chip Cookie Bites

Other Great Products:

ALDI-exclusive Simply Nature Grain Free Double Chocolate Cookie Bites

Bakeology Vanilla Chai Cookie Bites

You know you are gluten free

THE GUIDED BUYER.COM

When your bun costs more than the burger

Pizza Crust

2022 Annual Gluten Free Awards

1st Place Winner: MYBREAD Gluten Free Bakery Original Pizza Crusts

2nd Place Winner: BFree Foods Stone Baked Pizza Crust

3rd Place Winner: gf Jules Gluten Free Pizza Crust Mix

Runner Up: Cappello's Naked Pizza Crust

Other Great Products:

Schar Gluten Free Pizza Crust

Zeia Foods Gluten-Free Vegan Pizza Crust

Banza Plain Chickpea Pizza Crust

Rolls

2022 Annual Gluten Free Awards

1st Place Winner: Schar's Gluten Free Ciabatta Rolls

2nd Place Winner: Against the Grain Gourmet Rolls

3rd Place Winner: MYBREAD Gluten Free Bakery Original Dinner Rolls

Runner Up: Udi's Classic French Dinner Rolls

Other Great Products:

BFree Soft White Rolls

DELICIOUSLY SWEET, DECADENT, & GLUTEN-FREE

It's so good that you won't want to share it!

Tortilla

2022 Annual Gluten Free Awards

1st Place Winner: Food For Life Brown Rice Gluten Free Tortillas

2nd Place Winner: Mission Gluten Free Tortillas

3rd Place Winner: Siete Almond Flour Tortillas

Runner Up: Mission Soft Corn Tortilla

Other Great Products:

Tia Lupita Grain Free Tortillas

Toufayan Bakery Original Gluten Free Wraps / Tortillas

Wrap

2022 Annual Gluten Free Awards

1st Place Winner: BFree Foods Stone Baked Pita Bread

2nd Place Winner: ALDI-exclusive liveGfree Gluten Free Plain Wraps

3rd Place Winner: MYBREAD Gluten Free Bakery Original Flatbread Pitas

Runner Up: ALDI-exclusive liveGfree Gluten Free Spinach Wraps

Other Great Products:

BFree Foods Avocado Wrap

CELIAC SURVEY

We polled over 600 people with celiac disease with the intent to make you feel not so alone.

Do you have anxiety when eating out on a gluten free diet?

78% Yes

22% No

Presented by The 2022 Gluten Free Buyers Guide

YOU'RE NOT ALONE

34

Breakfast

Breakfast On-The-Go

2022 Annual Gluten Free Awards

1st Place Winner: Canyon Bakehouse Honey Whole Grain English Muffins

2nd Place Winner: Schär Cinnamon Raisin Bagels

3rd Place Winner: Goodie Girl Cookies® Blueberry Breakfast Biscuits

Runner Up: Bobo's Banana Peanut Butter Protein Bar

Other Great Products:

Bakery On Main Organic Probiotic Walnut Banana Premium Oatmeal

Glutino English Muffins

Cold Cereals

2022 Annual Gluten Free Awards

1st Place Winner: General Mills Cinnamon Chex

2nd Place Winner: Magic Spoon – Frosted

3rd Place Winner: General Mills Cheerios

Runner Up: Three Wishes Cocoa

Other Great Products:

General Mills Peanut Butter Chex

CELIAC SURVEY

We polled over 600 people with celiac disease
with the intent to make you feel not so alone.

Do you like to eat out
or at home?

85% Home

15% Out

Presented by The 2022 Gluten Free Buyers Guide

YOU'RE NOT ALONE

Donuts

2022 Annual Gluten Free Awards

1st Place Winner: Katz Gluten Free Glazed Donuts

2nd Place Winner: Katz Gluten Free Powdered Donuts

3rd Place Winner: ALDI-exclusive liveGfree Gluten Free Pumpkin Holiday Donuts

Runner Up: Kinnikinnick Gluten Free Cinnamon Sugar Donuts

Other Great Products:

Freedom Old Fashioned Glazed Gluten Free Donuts

ALDI-exclusive liveGfree Gluten Free Gingerbread Holiday Donuts

ALDI-exclusive liveGfree Gluten Free Cranberry Holiday Donuts

You know you are gluten free

THE GUIDED BUYER.COM

When you blow your paycheck at the grocery store

Frozen Pancake & Waffle Brands

2022 Annual Gluten Free Awards

1st Place Winner: Trader Joe's Gluten Free Toaster Waffles

2nd Place Winner: Birch Benders Gluten Free Toaster Waffles

3rd Place Winner: Van's Original Gluten Free Frozen Waffles

Runner Up: Vanilla Viking Waffles

Other Great Products:

Lopaus Point Wild Blueberry Waffles

Pancake and Waffle Mixes

2022 Annual Gluten Free Awards

1st Place Winner: Better Batter Pancake and Biscuit Mix

2nd Place Winner: gf Jules Pancake & Waffle Mix

3rd Place Winner: Kodiak Cakes Frontier Oat Gluten-Free Flapjack & Waffle Mix

Runner Up: King Arthur Gluten Free Pancake Mix

Other Great Products:

Betty Crocker Gluten Free Bisquick

CELIAC SURVEY

We polled over 600 people with celiac disease with the intent to make you feel not so alone.

Opinion: How long will it take before they find a cure for Celiac Disease?

Average: 38 More Years

YOU'RE NOT ALONE

Cookies, Snacks & Candy

Candy

2022 Annual Gluten Free Awards

1st Place Winner: Justin's Dark Chocolate Peanut Butter Crispy Cups

2nd Place Winner: Schär Twin Bar

3rd Place Winner: nib mor Tart Cherry Organic Dark Chocolate

Runner Up: No Whey! Milkless Crunchy

Other Great Products:

Yum Earth Strawberry Licorice

52

Chips

2022 Annual Gluten Free Awards

1st Place Winner: Siete Foods Ranch Grain Free Tortilla Chips

2nd Place Winner: ALDI-exclusive Simply Nature Blue Corn Tortilla Chips

3rd Place Winner: ALDI-exclusive Simply Nature Multigrain Tortilla Chips

Runner Up: Lay's Classic Chips

Other Great Products:

ALDI-exclusive Simply Nature Kettle Popcorn Chips

ALDI-exclusive Clancy's Veggie Chips

ALDI-exclusive Simply Nature Sea Salt Popcorn Chips

Late July Sea Salt & Lime

Crackers

2022 Annual Gluten Free Awards

1st Place Winner: Schär Gluten Free Table Crackers

2nd Place Winner: Mary's Gone Crackers Original

3rd Place Winner: Mary's Gone Crackers REAL Thin Sea Salt

Runner Up: Milton's Crispy Sea Salt Baked Crackers

Other Great Products:

Simple Mills Almond Flour Sea Salt Crackers

ALDI-exclusive Simply Nature Roasted Red Pepper Brown Rice Crackers

ALDI-exclusive Simply Nature Tomato & Basil Brown Rice Crackers

ALDI-exclusive Simply Nature Cinnamon Brown Sugar Butternut Squash Crackers

ALDI-exclusive Simply Nature Peppercorn Brown Rice Crackers

ALDI-exclusive Simply Nature Sea Salt Butternut Squash Crackers

CELIAC SURVEY

We polled over 600 people with celiac disease with the intent to make you feel not so alone.

Have you
ever knowingly cheated
on your gluten free diet?

31% Yes

69% No

Presented by The 2022 Gluten Free Buyers Guide

YOU'RE NOT ALONE

Granola

2022 Annual Gluten Free Awards

1st Place Winner: Bear Naked Maple Cinnamon Gluten Free Granola

2nd Place Winner: Bakery On Main Ancient Grain Cranberry Almond Maple Granola

3rd Place Winner: ALDI-exclusive Simply Nature Gluten Free Cranberry Cashew Granola

Runner Up: Safe + Fair The Birthday Cake Granola

Other Great Products:

Purely Elizabeth Original

You know you are gluten free

When you blame your
hangover on gluten

Jerky

2022 Annual Gluten Free Awards

1st Place Winner: Chomps Original Beef Jerky Sticks

2nd Place Winner: ALDI-exclsuive Simms Hickory Smoked Artisan Jerky

3rd Place Winner: The New Primal Sea Salt Beef Thins

Runner Up: Lorissa's Kitchen Korean BBQ jerky

Other Great Products:

Tillamook Zero Sugar Jerky

Munchies

2022 Annual Gluten Free Awards

1st Place Winner: Mary's Gone Crackers Super Seed Classic

2nd Place Winner: BOBO'S Strawberry Bites

3rd Place Winner: Bakery On Main Bakeshop Bliss White Chip Raspberry Swirl decadent Granola

Runner Up: ALDI-exclusive Fit & Active Cheddar Cheese Whole Grain Rice Snacks

Other Great Products:

ALDI-exclusive Fit & Active Caramel Whole Grain Rice Snacks

Pretzels

2022 Annual Gluten Free Awards

1st Place Winner: Snyder's of Hanover Gluten Free Pretzel Sticks

2nd Place Winner: Glutino Pretzel Twists

3rd Place Winner: Quinn Snacks Non-GMO and Gluten Free Pretzels, Classic Sea

Runner Up: Savor Street Grain Free Pretzel Twists - Gluten Free - Paleo Friendly

Other Great Products:

FitJoy Grain Free Pretzels, Gluten Free

Snack Bars

2022 Annual Gluten Free Awards

1st Place Winner: Schär Twin Bar

2nd Place Winner: BOBO'S Peanut Butter Chocolate Chip Protein Bars

3rd Place Winner: KIND Caramel Almond & Sea Salt

Runner Up: Bakery On Main Organic Oats & Honey Granola Bar

Other Great Products:

BeBOLD Bars Chocolate Chip Almond Butter

ALDI-exclusive Elevation Peanut Butter Cookie Bar

ALDI-exclusive Elevation Apple Pie Bar

LIDL Gluten Free High Protein Bar, Cookie Dough Flavored

Dessert

Ice Cream Cones

2022 Annual Gluten Free Awards

1st Place Winner: Joy Gluten-Free Sugar Ice Cream Cones

2nd Place Winner: Joy Gluten-Free Ice Cream Cones Cake Cups

3rd Place Winner: Sprouts Coconut Cones

Runner Up: Let's Do Gluten Free Ice Cream Cones

Other Great Products:

Let's Do Gluten Sugar Ice Cream Cones

CELIAC SURVEY

We polled over 600 people with celiac disease with the intent to make you feel not so alone.

Have you
ever knowingly cheated
on your gluten free diet?

31% Yes

69% No

Presented by The 2022 Gluten Free Buyers Guide

YOU'RE NOT ALONE

Pie Crust

2022 Annual Gluten Free Awards

1st Place Winner: King Arthur Gluten-Free Pie Crust

2nd Place Winner: Bob's Red Mill Gluten Free Pie Crust

3rd Place Winner: Midel Graham Cracker Crust

Runner Up: Trader Joes Gluten Free Pie Crust (frozen)

Other Great Products:

Wholly Wholesome Gluten Free Pie Crusts

Williams Sonoma Gluten-Free Pie Crust Mix

Cup4cup Gluten Free Pie Crust Mix

FLAX 4 LIFE
by Kasondra

Nutritious & Delicious Baked Goods

High in Fiber

Clean Ingredients

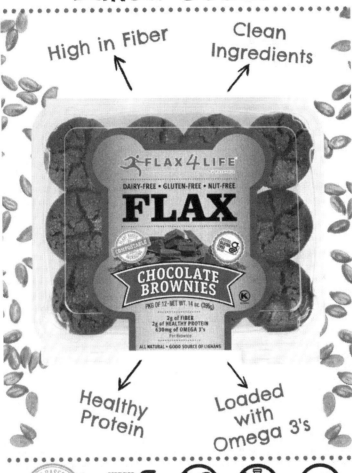

Healthy Protein

Loaded with Omega 3's

PLANT BASED COMPOSTABLE PACKAGING

CERTIFIED GLUTEN FREE
GFCO.ORG

NUT-FREE
*Except Coconut

DAIRY-FREE

KOSHER

Flax4Life.net

Ready Made Desserts

2022 Annual Gluten Free Awards

1st Place Winner: Katz Gluten Free Personal Size Cherry Pie

2nd Place Winner: Daiya New York Cheesecake Dairy Free & Gluten Free

3rd Place Winner: Better Bites BIRTHDAY DŌ BITES

Runner Up: Little Pie Company Gluten-Free Florida Key Lime Pie

Other Great Products:

Flax4Life Chocolate Brownies

FatBoy® Gluten-Free Ice Cream Cone

Beverages

Beer

2022 Annual Gluten Free Awards

1st Place Winner: Glutenberg

MICROBRASSERIE

Glutenberg

CRAFT BREWERY

— MTL.QC —

2nd Place Winner: Bards

3rd Place Winner: Ground Breaker Brewing

Runner Up: Redbridge

Other Great Beers:

Holidaily Brewing

Ghostfish Brewing

Dry Mixes

Bread Mixes

2022 Annual Gluten Free Awards

1st Place Winner: gfJules Bread Mix

2nd Place Winner: Pamela's Products Amazing Gluten-free Bread Mix

3rd Place Winner: Simple Mills Gluten Free Artisan Bread Mix

Runner Up: King Arthur Gluten-Free Bread and Pizza Mix

Other Great Products:

Bob's Red Mill Gluten Free Homemade Wonderful Bread Mix

CELIAC SURVEY

We polled over 600 people with celiac disease with the intent to make you feel not so alone.

After consuming gluten, do you have symptoms?

88% Yes Symptoms

11% No Symptoms

Presented by The 2022 Gluten Free Buyers Guide

YOU'RE NOT ALONE

Brownie Mixes

2022 Annual Gluten Free Awards

1st Place Winner: Krusteaz Gluten Free Double Chocolate Brownie Mix

2nd Place Winner: Betty Crocker Gluten Free Brownie Mix

3rd Place Winner: King Arthur Gluten Free Brownie Mix

Runner Up: Better Batter Fudge Brownie Mix

Other Great Products:

365 by Whole Foods Market, Brownie Gluten Free Mix

You know you are gluten free

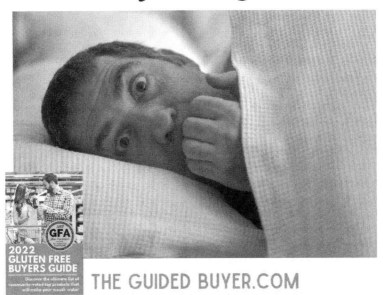

THE GUIDED BUYER.COM

When you have nightmares about eating regular food

Cake Mixes

2022 Annual Gluten Free Awards

1st Place Winner: King Arthur Gluten Free Confetti Cake Mix

2nd Place Winner: Namaste Yellow Cake Mix

3rd Place Winner: Better Batter Chocolate Cake Mix

Runner Up: Better Batter Yellow Cake Mix

Other Great Products:

Betty Crocker™ Gluten Free Yellow Cake Mix

CELIAC SURVEY

We polled over 600 people with celiac disease
with the intent to make you feel not so alone.

Do you eat something before you go out to eat?

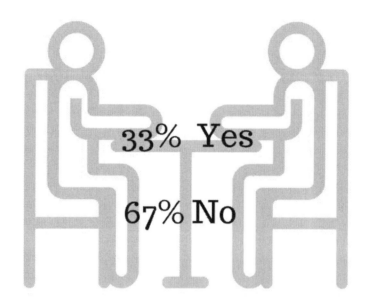

33% Yes

67% No

Presented by The 2022 Gluten Free Buyers Guide

YOU'RE NOT ALONE

Cookie Mixes

2022 Annual Gluten Free Awards

1st Place Winner: gfJules Cookie Mix

2nd Place Winner: 365 by Whole Foods Market, Chocolate Chip Gluten Free Cookie Mix

3rd Place Winner: Meli's Monster Gluten Free Cookies (Original)

Runner Up: Good Dees Butter Pecan Cookie Mix, Low Carb & Gluten Free

Other Great Products:

Betty Crocker Gluten Free Chocolate Chip Cookie Mix

CELIAC SURVEY

We polled over 600 people with celiac disease
with the intent to make you feel not so alone.

Do you
have other family with
Celiac Disease?

47% Yes

53% No

Presented by The 2022 Gluten Free Buyers Guide

YOU'RE NOT ALONE

Cornbread Mixes

2022 Annual Gluten Free Awards

1st Place Winner: Krusteaz Gluten Free Honey Cornbread Mix

2nd Place Winner: gfJules Cornbread Mix

3rd Place Winner: Cup4Cup Gluten Free Cornbread Mix

Runner Up: ALDI-exclusive liveGfree Gluten Free Cornbread Mix

Other Great Products:

Bob's Red Mill Cornbread Mix

Flours

2022 Annual Gluten Free Awards

1st Place Winner: gfJules All Purpose Gluten Free Flour

2nd Place Winner: Pamela's Products Gluten Free All Purpose Flour Blend

3rd Place Winner: Bob's Red Mill 1:1 Gluten Free Flour

Runner Up: Better Batter Artisan Baker's Blend

Other Great Products:

King Arthur Measure for Measure Gluten Free Flour

ALDI-exclusive Baker's Corner Almond Flour

Muffin Mixes

2022 Annual Gluten Free Awards

1st Place Winner: Simple Mills Almond Flour Gluten Free Chocolate Cake Muffin Mix

2nd Place Winner: gf Jules Muffin Mix

3rd Place Winner: King Arthur Gluten Free Muffin Mix

Runner Up: Krusteaz Gluten Free Blueberry Muffin Mix

Other Great Products:

Lakanto Gluten Free Banana Nut Muffin and Bread Mix

Frozen Foods

Frozen Food

2022 Annual Gluten Free Awards

1st Place Winner: Evol Fire Grilled Steak Bowl

2nd Place Winner: LIDL Frozen Gluten Free Fish Sticks

3rd Place Winner: Feel Good Foods Vegetable Potstickers

Runner Up: ALDI-exclusive Whole & Simple Shrimp & Asparagus Single Serves

Other Great Products:

ALDI-exclusive Whole & Simple Shrimp & Quinoa Single Serves

Amy's Gluten Free Mac and Cheese

CELIAC SURVEY

We polled over 600 people with celiac disease with the intent to make you feel not so alone.

At work, are you the only one with Celiac Disease?

78% Yes

22% No

YOU'RE NOT ALONE

Frozen Meals

2022 Annual Gluten Free Awards

1st Place Winner: Udi's Italian Sausage Lasagna Frozen Entreé

2nd Place Winner: Amy's Gluten Free Chinese Noodles & Veggies

3rd Place Winner: Primal Kitchen Chicken Pesto Bowl

Runner Up: ALDI-exclusive liveGfree General Tso's Chicken

Other Great Products:

Blake's Gluten Free Chicken Pot Pie

Frozen Pizza Brands

2022 Annual Gluten Free Awards

1st Place Winner: Freschetta Gluten Free Pepperoni Pizza

2nd Place Winner: Against the Grain Pepperoni Pizza

3rd Place Winner: ALDI-exclusive Mama Cozzi's Pizza Kitchen Cauliflower Crust Margherita Pizza

Runner Up: California Pizza Kitchen Gluten Free Pizza BBQ Chicken

Other Great Products:

ALDI-exclusive Mama Cozzi's Pizza Kitchen Cauliflower Crust Cheese Pizza

ALDI-exclusive Mama Cozzi's Pizza Kitchen Roasted Vegetable Cauliflower Pizza

CELIAC SURVEY

We polled over 600 people with celiac disease
with the intent to make you feel not so alone.

Do you drink gluten removed beer or stick to gluten free beers?

84% Gluten Free Only

6% Gluten Removed

10% Both

Presented by The 2022 Gluten Free Buyers Guide

YOU'RE NOT ALONE

Health & Beauty

Cosmetic Brands

2022 Annual Gluten Free Awards

1st Place Winner: Red Apple Lipstick

2nd Place Winner: Arbonne

3rd Place Winner: Honeybee Gardens

Runner Up: Gabriel Cosmetics

GABRIEL

Other Great Products:

Zuzu Luxe

ZUZU LUXE

We've got that ooey gooey gluten-free.

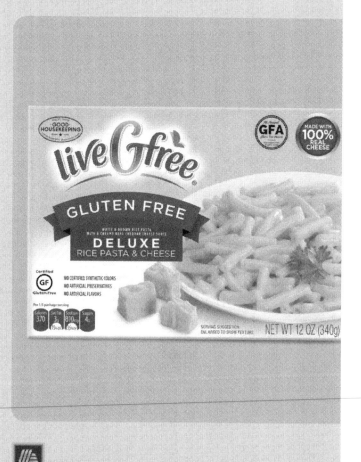

Magazine & Books

Books

2022 Annual Gluten Free Awards

1st Place Winner: The First Year: Celiac Disease and Living Gluten-Free: An Essential Guide for the Newly Diagnosed: Jules Shepard

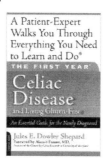

2nd Place Winner: Dear Gluten, It's Not Me, It's You: How to Survive Without Gluten and Restore Your Health from Celiac Disease or Gluten Sensitivity by Jenny Levine Finke and Dr. Tom O'Bryan

3rd Place Winner: I'm a Gluten-Sniffing Service Dog by Michal Babay (Author), Ela Smietanka (Illustrator)

Runner Up: Gluten Freedom: The Nation's Leading Expert Offers the Essential Guide to a Healthy, Gluten-Free Lifestyle by Alessio Fasano (Author), Susie Flaherty (Contributor)

Other Great Books:

Gluten Is My Bitch: Rants, Recipes, and Ridiculousness for the Gluten-Free

Living Gluten-Free For Dummies

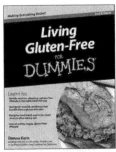

CELIAC SURVEY

We polled over 600 people with celiac disease with the intent to make you feel not so alone.

Do you have a dedicated gluten free toaster in your kitchen?

72% Yes

28% No

Presented by The 2022 Gluten Free Buyers Guide

YOU'RE NOT ALONE

Children's Books

2022 Annual Gluten Free Awards

1st Place Winner: Everyone's Got Something: My First Year with Celiac Disease by Hallie Rose Katzman, Rayna Mae Katzman

2nd Place Winner: I'm a Gluten-Sniffing Service Dog by Michal Babay (Author), Ela Smietanka (Illustrator)

3rd Place Winner: Eat Like a Dinosaur: Recipe & Guidebook for Gluten-free Kids by Paleo Parents and Elana Amsterdam

Runner Up: My Perfect Cupcake: A Recipe for Thriving with Food Allergies (The Fearless Food Allergy Friends) by Rebecca Greene and Rebecca Sinclair

Other Great Books:

Gluten Free is Part of Me by Laurie Oestreich

Cookbooks

2022 Annual Gluten Free Awards

1st Place Winner: How to Make Anything Gluten-Free: Over 100 recipes for everything from home comforts to fakeaways, cakes to dessert, brunch to bread! by Becky Excell

2nd Place Winner: Nearly Normal Cooking For Gluten-Free Eating: A Fresh Approach to Cooking and Living Without Wheat or Gluten by Jules E. D. Shepard and Alessio Fasano

3rd Place Winner: Cook Once, Eat All Week: 26 Weeks of Gluten-Free, Affordable Meal Prep to Preserve Your Time & Sanity by Cassy Joy Garcia

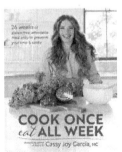

Runner Up: Flavcity's 5 Ingredient Meals: 50 Easy & Tasty Recipes Using the Best Ingredients from the Grocery Store (Heart Healthy Budget Cooking) by Bobby Parrish & Dessi Parrish

Other Great Cookbooks:

The Defined Dish: Whole30 Endorsed, Healthy and Wholesome Weeknight Recipes Hardcover by Alex Snodgrass

Gluten-Free on a Shoestring: 125 Easy Recipes for Eating Well on the Cheap by Nicole Hunn

You know you are gluten free

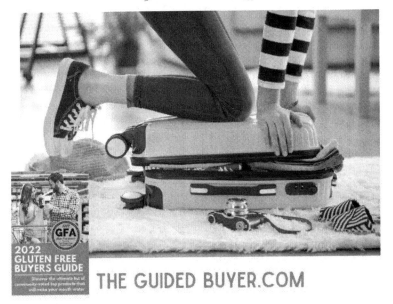

THE GUIDED BUYER.COM

When you pack more food than clothes

Magazines

2022 Annual Gluten Free Awards

1st Place Winner: Simply Gluten Free

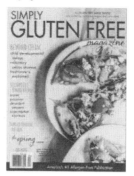

2nd Place Winner: GFF Magazine

3rd Place Winner: Allergic Living

CELIAC SURVEY

We polled over 600 people with celiac disease
with the intent to make you feel not so alone.

Do you
try to keep your diagnosis
a secret or do you share
your story?

58% Share
42% It depends
0% Keep it secret

Presented by The 2022 Gluten Free Buyers Guide

YOU'RE NOT ALONE

Media

Blogs & Websites

2022 Annual Gluten Free Awards

1st Place Winner: GFJules.com

2nd Place Winner: GlutenFreeFollowMe.com

3rd Place Winner: WhatTheForkFoodBlog.com

Runner Up: GlutenFreeOnAShoestring.com

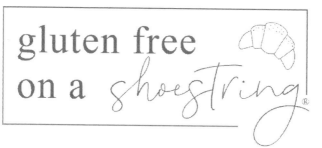

Other Great Blogs & Websites:

Healthy GF Family

Celiac Project

The Paleo Mom

Stayglutenfree.com

Gluten Free Globetrotter

The Gluten Free Travelers

Cure Celiac Disease.org

Gluten Free RN

Living Freely Gluten Free

Mobile Apps

2022 Annual Gluten Free Awards

1st Place Winner: Find Me Gluten Free

2nd Place Winner: The Gluten Free Scanner

3rd Place Winner: Gluten Dude Mobile App

Runner Up: Spokin

Other Great Apps:

Spoonful

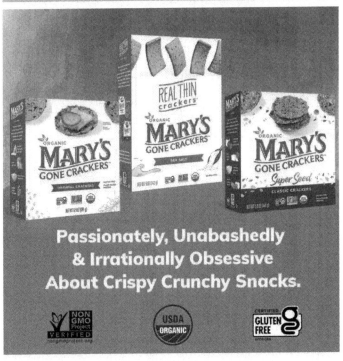

130

Nonprofits

2022 Annual Gluten Free Awards

1st Place Winner: Celiac Disease Foundation (CDF)

2nd Place Winner: Gluten Intolerance Group of North America (GIG)

3rd Place Winner: Beyond Celiac

Runner Up: National Celiac Organization

Online Resources

2022 Annual Gluten Free Awards

1st Place Winner: Celiac.org

2nd Place Winner: GlutenFreeWatchDog.org

3rd Place Winner: Beyondceliac.org

Runner Up: Glutenfreefollowme.com

Other Great Resources:

gfJules.com

VOTED #1 GLUTEN FREE FLOUR & MIXES
IN 2020 FOR THE 4TH TIME!

CELIAC SURVEY

We polled over 600 people with celiac disease with the intent to make you feel not so alone.

Does your family support your gluten free lifestyle?

95% Yes

5% No

Presented by The 2022 Gluten Free Buyers Guide

YOU'RE NOT ALONE

Podcasts

2022 Annual Gluten Free Awards

1st Place Winner: Gluten Free You & Me

2nd Place Winner: The Celiac Project Podcast

3rd Place Winner: Celiac Straight Talk by Beyond Celiac

Runner Up: Gluten Free New with Andrea Tucker

Other Great Podcasts:

Celiac & Gluten Free Living with Deb

You know you are gluten free

THE GUIDED BUYER.COM

When regular bread gets set on your gluten free order

Other

Comfort Foods

2022 Annual Gluten Free Awards

1st Place Winner: Amy's Gluten Free Rice Mac & Cheese

2nd Place Winner: MYBREAD Gluten Free Bakery Original Soft Breadsticks

3rd Place Winner: Feel Good Foods Three Cheese Mac & Cheese Bites

Runner Up: Jolly Feel Good Foods Mozzarella Sticks

Other Great Products:

Kraft Gluten Free Mac and Cheese

Gluten Free Pizza (Refrigerated)

2022 Annual Gluten Free Awards

1st Place Winner: ALDI-exclusive Mama Cozzi's Pizza Kitchen 12" Gluten Free Pepperoni Deli Pizza

2nd Place Winner: ALDI-exclusive Mama Cozzi's Pizza Kitchen 12" Gluten Free Cheese Deli Pizza

3rd Place Winner: ALDI-exclusive Mama Cozzi's Pizza Kitchen 12" Cauliflower Crust Pepperoni Deli Pizza

Runner Up: ALDI-exclusive Mama Cozzi's Pizza Kitchen 12" Cauliflower Crust Cheese Deli Pizza

ALDI-exclusive Mama Cozzi's Pizza Kitchen 12" Cauliflower Crust Veggie Deli Pizza

CELIAC SURVEY

We polled over 600 people with celiac disease
with the intent to make you feel not so alone.

Have you gained or lost weight on a gluten free diet?

66% Gained weight

34% Lost weight

Presented by The 2022 Gluten Free Buyers Guide

YOU'RE NOT ALONE

New Products

2022 Annual Gluten Free Awards

1st Place Winner: Bakery On Main Bakeshop Bliss Monster Cookie Decadent Granola

2nd Place Winner: imPASTA! Foods Ready-to-eat spaghetti squash

3rd Place Winner: Nabisco Gluten Free Oreos

Runner Up: Jolly Feel Good Foods Deep Dish Pizza

Other Great Products:

LIDL Vegan Quinoa Salad, Zucchini and Onion Sauce

Purecane™ Baking Sweetener

Feel Good Foods Mozzarella Sticks

CELIAC SURVEY

We polled over 600 people with celiac disease with the intent to make you feel not so alone.

What food do you miss the most?

#1 Take Out Pizza

#2 Pastries

#3 Fried Chicken

#4 Chinese Food

Presented by The 2022 Gluten Free Buyers Guide

YOU'RE NOT ALONE

Pasta, Sides, Soup & Sauces

Macaroni and Cheese

2022 Annual Gluten Free Awards

1st Place Winner: Kraft Gluten Free Macaroni & Cheese

2nd Place Winner: ALDI-exclusive liveGfree Gluten Free Deluxe Macaroni & Cheese

3rd Place Winner: Amy's Gluten Free Macaroni & Cheese

Runner Up: LIDL Gluten Free Rice Shells & Cheese

Other Great Products:

Trader Joe's Frozen Gluten Free Mac & Cheese

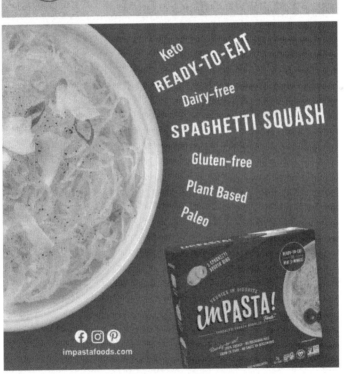

Pastas

2022 Annual Gluten Free Awards

1st Place Winner: CAULIPOWER Linguine Cauliflower Pasta

2nd Place Winner: Barilla Spaghetti

3rd Place Winner: Le Veneziane Fettucce

Runner Up: Jovial Tagliatelle

Other Great Products:

ALDI-exclusive Simply Nature Chickpea Penne

ALDI-exclusive Simply Nature Red Lentil Rotini

Tinkyada Brown Rice Penne

Condiments

2022 Annual Gluten Free Awards

1st Place Winner: San-J Hoisin Sauce

2nd Place Winner: Mike's Hot Honey

3rd Place Winner: Noble Made by The New Primal Tomato Ketchup

Runner Up: Trader Joe's Coconut Aminos

Other Great Products:

San-J Organic Tamari Soy Sauce

Dips and Spreads

2022 Annual Gluten Free Awards

1st Place Winner: Justin's Chocolate Hazelnut and Almond Butter

2nd Place Winner: Siete Dairy Free Cashew Queso, Spicy Blanco

3rd Place Winner: Skinnygirl Sugar Free Preserves, Apricot Mimosa

Runnor Up: Sahra Hummus

Other Great Products:

Mikes Hot Honey

Dressing

2022 Annual Gluten Free Awards

1st Place Winner: Hidden Valley The Original Ranch Plant Powered, Gluten Free & Dairy Free Ranch Salad Dressing

2nd Place Winner: Dress It Up Dressing - Sesame Tahini Gluten Free Salad Dressing and Marinade

3rd Place Winner: Wu Japanese Gluten Free Ginger Dressing

Runner Up: Ken's Steak House Chunky Blue Cheese

Other Great Products:

Yo Mama's Foods American Ranch

CELIAC SURVEY

We polled over 600 people with celiac disease
with the intent to make you feel not so alone.

Do you pack gluten free food in your baggage when traveling?

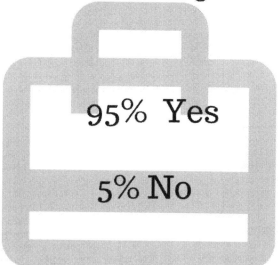

95% Yes

5% No

Presented by The 2022 Gluten Free Buyers Guide

YOU'RE NOT ALONE

Sauces

2022 Annual Gluten Free Awards

1st Place Winner: San-J Organic Tamari Soy Sauce

2nd Place Winner: ALDI-exclusive Specially Selected Italian Herb Pasta Sauce

3rd Place Winner: Kevin's Natural Foods Teriyaki Sauce - Keto, Gluten Free & Paleo Simmer Sauce

Runner Up: ALDI-exclusive Specially Selected Four Cheese Pasta Sauce

Other Great Products:

ALDI-exclusive Specially Selected Sensitive Recipe Pasta Sauce

Trader Joe's Organic Coconut Aminos

CELIAC SURVEY

We polled over 600 people with celiac disease with the intent to make you feel not so alone.

Do you think the celebrity / Hollywood gluten free trend helped or hurt those with Celiac Disease?

52% Hurt

48% Helped

Presented by The 2022 Gluten Free Buyers Guide

YOU'RE NOT ALONE

Soup

2022 Annual Gluten Free Awards

1st Place Winner: Thai Kitchen Instant Rice Noodle Soup - Gluten Free Ramen

2nd Place Winner: Progresso Gluten Free Homestyle Chicken Noodle

3rd Place Winner: Oma's Own Organic Instant Rice Ramen Noodle Cups, no Chicken Noodle - Gluten Free

Runner Up: Wild Zora Instant Lemon Chicken with Vegetables

Other Great Products:

Mr. Lee's Hong Kong Street-Style Beef Rice Noodle Soup

CELIAC SURVEY

We polled over 600 people with celiac disease with the intent to make you feel not so alone.

Have people made fun of the gluten free diet in front of you?

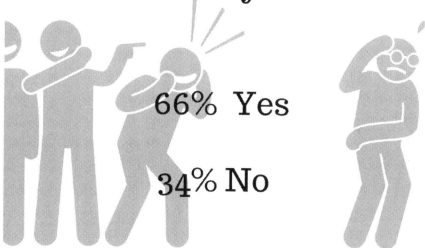

66% Yes

34% No

Presented by The 2022 Gluten Free Buyers Guide

YOU'RE NOT ALONE

Stuffing

2022 Annual Gluten Free Awards

1st Place Winner: Aleia's Best. Taste. Ever. Savory Stuffing

2nd Place Winner: Three Bakers Herb Seasoned Whole Grain Cubed Stuffing

3rd Place Winner: Olivia's Croutons - Rosemary & Sage Stuffing

Runner Up: Aleia's Best. Taste. Ever. Plain Stuffing

Other Great Products:

Trader Joes Gluten Free Stuffing Mix

Personalities

Best Gluten Free Personality

2022 Annual Gluten Free Awards

1st Place Winner: Jules Shepard

2nd Place Winner: Jackie Aanonsen McEwan

3rd Place Winner: Sharon Lachendro

Runner Up: Michael Frolichstein

Other great gluten free people:

Gluten Dude

Erica Dermer

Andrea Tucker

Patrick Auger

Erin Smith

Jackie McEwan

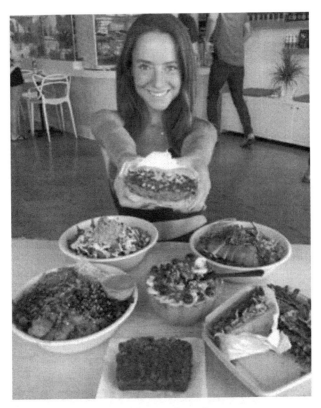

How long have you been gluten free?

8+ years

Do you have any other dietary restrictions?

Just gluten

What has been your biggest challenge thus far?

My biggest challenge was when I found out that I had to follow a gluten-free diet. I was completely overwhelmed. I did not even know what gluten was! I had to figure out what foods I could eat, what foods I had to avoid, and the nuances in between. I wished I had a go-to guide to tell me all I needed to know about following a gluten-free diet. This manual did not yet exist, so I did a ton of research and learned how to maneuver being gluten-free at restaurants and in my own kitchen.

In March 2014, I started to post about some of the gluten-free foods I was eating on Instagram. Surprisingly to me, my posts were met with great reception. People I had never met were asking me for more tips on gluten-free friendly eateries, products, and recipes, and I was more than happy to continue to make these discoveries. I was getting so many questions that I knew I needed to put all this information in one place rather than just Instagram.

In September 2014, I taught myself how to make a website, and I launched glutenfreefollowme.com! I wish I had something like Gluten Free Follow Me to guide me through my new gluten-free diet eight years ago, but I am glad I can be a guide for others now! At the time, going gluten-free seemed like the worst thing ever. However, I am grateful for it now. Knowledge is power, and I am healthier because of it. Going gluten-free led me to start Gluten Free Follow Me. If I had not become gluten-free, I would probably still be working in finance in New York City. My quest to find gluten-free foods developed into a full-time passion, and I could not be happier with how it all turned out!

Where is your favorite place to eat?

I have many favorites! A few of my faves are: Posh Pop Bakeshop in NYC, Vibe Organic Kitchen in Newport Beach, and Petunia's Pies & Pastries in Portland. Many more on glutenfreefollowme.com/restaurants :)

Do you have any gluten related pet peeves?

When someone says that they could never give up gluten. When you have to, yes you can! And honestly, it's not that hard, especially nowadays. There are so many amazing options.

How has the Covid quarantine changed your diet habits?

I can't say that it has! I still eat fairly balanced with lots of fruits and veggies, and my fair share of chocolate, baked goods, and sweets :)

Do you have a gluten horror story?

Back when I was working in NYC, I went out to lunch at a restaurant that is now closed. I told the hostess, manager, and waitress that I was gluten-free. They went through the menu with me and told me which options were safe for me to eat. I ended up ordering the nachos as an appetizer. I had just taken my first bite of the nachos when the manager ran over to tell me that the nachos were not actually gluten-free. The chips had cross contamination in the fryer. I couldn't believe it! It was even more frustrating because I had asked the right questions. Thankfully, something like this hasn't happened to me again.

What has been the biggest change since you became gluten free?

Every year, it becomes easier to follow a gluten-free diet! It's more straightforward to find gluten-free foods. Supermarkets and stores now have gluten-free sections, and food labeling has gotten better. Products market themselves to the gluten-free consumer. Some brands have even modified their ingredients in order to make their products gluten-free. The restaurant scene has become more sensitive to people who follow a gluten-free diet. Some restaurants have menus that indicate which items are gluten-free, and this definitely wasn't the case seven years ago. Waiters are usually well-versed in how to accommodate dietary needs, unlike a few years ago when the majority of waiters didn't even know what gluten was.

In ten years, a gluten free diet will be···

Even more widespread. I see the gluten-free world continuing down the path of increased awareness. I've eaten at 75 completely gluten-free eateries, and I expect to see even more 100% gluten-free eateries in the future. I predict that the number of people who go gluten-free will keep on multiplying. After all, gluten-free food truly tastes good now, and it's a healthier way to live.

What is the best advice you received?

Make something people want.

What is the best way for people to connect with you?

Instagram: @glutenfree.followme

Twitter: @glutenfreefm

Facebook: Gluten Free Follow Me

Blog: glutenfreefollowme.com

CELIAC SURVEY

We polled over 600 people with celiac disease
with the intent to make you feel not so alone.

Do you feel alone living the gluten free lifestyle?

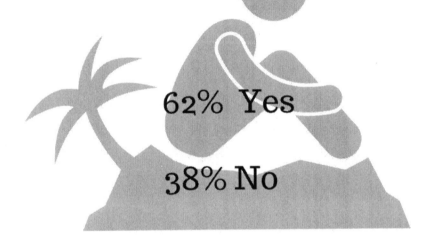

62% Yes

38% No

Presented by The 2022 Gluten Free Buyers Guide

YOU'RE NOT ALONE

Jules Shepard

How long have you been gluten free?

21 years!

Do you have any other dietary restrictions?

No dairy, mostly vegan and I don't do any meat.

What has been your biggest challenge thus far?

Personally, my challenge has just been if I want to eat out. I can really make anything I want for myself and my family at home, so for travel or socializing with friends at a restaurant, it can be a bit challenging, awkward and sometimes very stressful to put my trust in a restaurant instead.

Where is your favorite place to eat?

Haha ... speaking of trusting someone else! My favorite place to eat besides home (!) is no longer open. It was one of the places I looked forward to visiting when I traveled out west for gluten-free shows or to see friends, and I learned that due to the pandemic, it closed its doors. I was so sad to learn of its demise, as well as that of so many other dedicated gluten free restaurants around the country. I truly hope that we'll see a return of dedicated GF restaurants again one day once the country recovers.

Do you have any gluten related pet peeves?

Doesn't everyone?!

It still annoys me when people think that gluten is a fad or that being gluten free is some kind of choice for us. It also annoys me that there are so many food companies out there who still make bad gluten free food! It's like they don't eat their own products!! Cheap ingredients made bad food -- it's a pretty simple concept. But the end result is that gluten free food still has a bad name because of it. Gluten free food can be super delicious and people need to know that, but they have to be exposed to the right ingredients and products, so there's still a lot of work to be done.

How has the Covid quarantine changed your diet habits?

It hasn't changed my habits much, since we hardly ever ate out before. But we actually have tried to order take out MORE than we did before just to help restaurants stay in business. So I guess in that way it has changed our habits a bit, but there aren't a lot of gluten free restaurant options near us, so I suppose the ones nearby are getting more used to seeing our name pop up on their caller ID!

Do you have a gluten horror story?

How many do you want? I already told you I've been gluten free for 21 years, so that's a lot of time for horror stories! I have plenty to have accumulated during that time, but also before I was diagnosed and during the 10 years I was still eating gluten before I was diagnosed and was so sick. Gluten and I really don't get along very well at all! Pretty much anyone reading this can think on their own horror stories and I've been right there with you. If you want some more specifics, I outline several in my book, The First Year: Celiac Disease and Living Gluten Free.

What has been the biggest change since you became gluten free?

People in the general population actually have heard of gluten and celiac disease! When I was diagnosed, no one (including myself) had even heard of gluten. So there have been many, many changes. There are products on the market that are made FOR people eating gluten free, products are labeled and certified gluten free, there are gluten free menus, there are blood tests for celiac disease, there is a genetic test for celiac disease ... so many changes!

In ten years, a gluten free diet will be···

Completely mainstream.

What is the best advice you received?

I didn't. There was no one to give me advice when I was told I had to go gluten free. Literally, my doctor told me I had celiac disease and couldn't eat gluten, and then he said he thought it was in bread, but wasn't sure what it was. There were no nutritionists at the time to help me, no internet resources, no books to speak of ... it was a real wasteland of information. I ate Rice Krispies cereal until I figured out for myself that malt flavoring contained barley which also contained gluten. Then I ate Peppermint Patties because I thought they didn't have any gluten in them. And rice. I ate lots of rice. It was a dark time for me! (Don't worry, I finally figured it out!)

What is the best way for people to connect with you?

@gfJules on FB, IG & Pinterest and @THEgfJules on Twitter or through my blog gfJules.com.

CELIAC SURVEY

We polled over 600 people with celiac disease
with the intent to make you feel not so alone.

Should we be charged
extra for a gluten free bun?

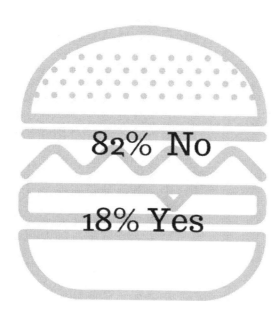

82% No

18% Yes

Presented by The 2022 Gluten Free Buyers Guide

YOU'RE NOT ALONE

Erica Dermer

How long have you been gluten free?

10-ish years! There were a few years of on and off diagnoses while I was waiting on a celiac disease true diagnosis!

Do you have any other dietary restrictions?

I can't eat beef - haven't had it in 12 or so years. I've cut out dairy for about 5-6 years, and eggs on and off for years. I now eat baked eggs (like eggs in bread).

What has been your biggest challenge thus far?

Fighting the misinformation of the internet! Unfortunately, too many still view gluten free as a "diet to try" when in reality it's a medical diet that should be given by a medical professional after a celiac disease screening.

Where is your favorite place to eat?

We're so lucky to have so many great dedicated gluten-free restaurants and bakeries here in Phoenix, and gluten-free friendly restaurants. I don't have a favorite - I just love to eat!

Do you have any gluten related pet peeves?

Brands that don't have easily accessible information on their website or social media about how their product is made and how/where they source their ingredients.

How has the Covid quarantine changed your diet habits?

I have been buying a lot more products online and in bulk! However, you have to be really careful to not try new products in bulk - or else you have a LOT of something you don't like!

Do you have a gluten horror story?

Most of the "horror stories" revolve around front of the house servers or managers that don't understand the seriousness of making a restaurant item safe for those with celiac, after claiming it is "gluten free."

What has been the biggest change since you became gluten free?

We are so lucky - in 2020 we have so many great gluten-free products out there. Seriously, name a product and we have a gluten-free replacement out there. We've grown so much!

In ten years, a gluten free diet will be···

Hopefully better understood as a medically-necessary diet.

What is the best advice you received?

It will get easier, it just takes time.

What is the best way for people to connect with you?

Hit me up on social media or email! I love to chat about celiac disease!

CELIAC SURVEY

We polled over 600 people with celiac disease with the intent to make you feel not so alone.

Do you attend any celiac support group meetings?

32% Yes

68% No

Presented by The 2022 Gluten Free Buyers Guide

YOU'RE NOT ALONE

Michael Frolichstein

How long have you been gluten free?

11 years

Do you have any other dietary restrictions?

No

What has been your biggest challenge thus far?

Normally, my biggest challenge would be the social gatherings which include food, but during this time of social distancing, I'm finding that I am more anxious to order food from restaurants for take-out. I am wary of getting glutened.

Where is your favorite place to eat?

I have a few, but my favorite would be Wildfire. It is a classic steakhouse style restaurant with a full gluten free menu the size of their original, and excellent protocols in place so they consistently "do it right." A nice touch is that they have our name in their system and just grab gluten free menus without us needing to ask. Plus, my wife and daughters love it, too!

Do you have any gluten related pet peeves?

My biggest pet peeve is that so many people can't wrap their minds around cross contamination. I still get strange looks and eye rolls when avoiding gluten free foods in certain situations. With The Celiac Project, I'm all about educating others, but sometimes in these personal situations I'm just frustrated and want to relax.

How has the Covid quarantine changed your diet habits?

Luckily, my wife, Ellen, is a great cook and is constantly making all of the favorite meals and treats that our family loves. It has brought comfort during this time of uncertainty. Also, there have been many great guests on the podcast who have given us tips on how to have unique food experiences at home, which we are having fun experimenting with.

Do you have a gluten horror story?

Unfortunately, yes! I guess we all have at least one, and when I tell this story around my kids, they just cringe. We were making tacos and using a brand of tortillas that we thought at the time only made the corn variety. Midway through dinner my daughter, Jessica, also a celiac, commented on the taste and texture being so amazing and different than what she was used to. My wife and my eyes met in horror. I ran to the kitchen, read the package and they were wheat tortillas. I was in total disbelief at the mistake and by then it was too late. I had one of the most terrible nights of my life. So sick as a dog and I even passed out on the floor. It was the only time, to my knowledge, in the past 11 years that I knowingly consumed a gluten containing product. It was a great reminder to always double and triple check the ingredients and make no assumptions.

What has been the biggest change since you became gluten free?

Since becoming gluten free 11 years ago, the level of daily brain fog, illness, and anxiety that permeated my life since childhood dissipated, and the renewed sense of how I could redefine myself moving forward was liberating. Becoming gluten free changed more than my health, it changed the course of my life, inspiring me to start The Celiac Project-- my documentary and podcast, helping to raise awareness and bring our community together. I am very grateful for that!

In ten years, a gluten free diet will be...

...not considered a fad. My fear is that we might lose some products and restaurants, but the ones that remain will be more consistently trustworthy to the celiac and gluten intolerant community. There is also a real possibility that in ten years there will be a treatment that will hopefully allow us to not worry about cross contamination, which would be a true game-changer.

What is the best advice you received?

Stay the course. Although some people can feel better after just a couple of weeks on a gluten free diet, the majority of us take much longer to heal their gut and have their symptoms subside. This takes patience, being good to yourself emotionally when you're having a tough time because getting better is not always a straight line. Finding a good support system is also important so you don't feel alone.

What is the best way for people to connect with you?

If you would like to interact with me in a more personal way, go to www.celiacproject.com and join our Patreon #TCP Inner Circle where you can participate in a monthly live hangout with me, my podcast co-host, Cam Weiner, and our fellow community as we talk all things celiac and gluten free in an open, supportive, and positive forum. You can also email me at info@celiacproject.com and find me on Facebook, twitter or instagram @celiacproject

CELIAC SURVEY

We polled over 600 people with celiac disease with the intent to make you feel not so alone.

Is it harder to date others when you are on a gluten free diet?

63% Yes

37% No

Presented by The 2022 Gluten Free Buyers Guide

YOU'RE NOT ALONE

Andrea Tucker

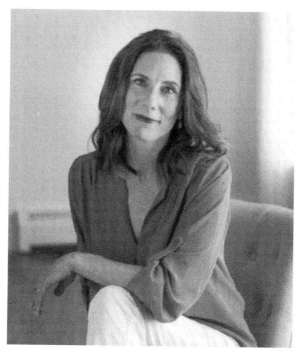

How long have you been gluten free?

10 years

Do you have any other dietary restrictions?

No

What has been your biggest challenge thus far?

Finding community and vetted sources of information. That was the motivation for starting my podcast, The Gluten Free News.

Where is your favorite place to eat?

HeartBeet Kitchen in Westmont, NJ

Do you have any gluten related pet peeves?

Products labeled gluten free that aren't.

How has the Covid quarantine changed your diet habits?

We are now eating every day at home with occasional take out from safe eateries.

Do you have a gluten horror story?

After many conversations at a small restaurant, my gluten free daughter found a piece of spaghetti in her salad. Needless to say, I let the manager know and have stayed far away from the establishment.

What has been the biggest change since you became gluten free?

The quality and quantity of gluten free products. The bread has gotten so much better too!

In ten years, a gluten free diet will be···

Well- understood and taken seriously.

What is the best advice you received?

To have a 504 plan for my daughter. It's an excellent tool for educating faculty and staff that follows her from year to year.

What is the best way for people to connect with you?

Social Media:

IG: baltimoreglutenfree FB: balimoreglutenfree Twitter: baltgf

The only ingredients we skipped, were gluten.

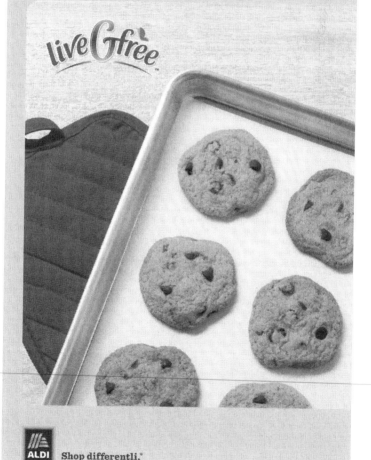

Gluten Free Product Registration

By submitting your products into The Gluten Free Awards (GFA), you are automatically entering products into the Annual Gluten Free Buyers Guide. There are only 10 slots available in each category and we limit brands to 3 submissions per category. If you are a marketer representing multiple brands, this typically will not apply. Slots can fill quickly so we recommend submitting your registration ASAP. The absolute deadline for registration is August 22nd however, we cannot guarantee you that the category is already full.

"How do I get into the Gluten Free Awards?"

How it works:

1. Fill out the registration form by adding the quantities and product names.

(A free half page ad is given for every 5 products or full-page ad for 10 products.)

2. If wanted, add additional ad space to registration.

3. Email the registration form to Jayme@GlutenFreeBuyersGuide.com

4. We will follow up with a confirmation and invoice.

If you have any questions call customer support at 828-455-9734

"Wait, I have tons of questions still"

Most common questions:

Q: I am having a hard time understanding how to submit or products.

A: Using this Registration Form will help. If lost, don't hesitate to call or email. 828-455-9734

Q: What are the image specs you need?

A: Our graphic team just needs images that are PDF, JPEG or PNG at 300 dpi or greater. The team will normally resize images based on the publishing media. Normally the product pictures and descriptions from your website will work just fine.

Full Page Ad Size 384 by 576 px

Half Page Ad Size 384 by 288 px

Q: Is there a word count for product descriptions?

A: No, we normally don't use product descriptions just product names and images.

Q: If we submit 10 products do, we get 1 free full-page ad and 2 free half page ads?

A: Sorry, please choose one or the other. You can always purchase additional ad space.

Q: Can we run a full-page ad without entering the awards program?

A: Yes.

Q: Do we need to send you product samples?

A: No. The gluten-free community votes for your products.

Q: Will we be in the guide if we don't win an award?

A: Yes, all products submitted will be visible as nominees.

Q: Can we use the GFA Nominee and Winner Badge on our product packaging, website and other related media?

A: Yes, we highly recommend using the badges to differentiate your products from the rest. If you happen to need higher resolution images don't hesitate to ask. Read our media terms here.

Need to talk about your order or have questions? Give us a call.

828-455-9734

or email

Josh@GlutenFreeBuyersGuide.com

From our family to yours, have a happy and healthy gluten free lifestyle.

The Schieffer Family

Josh (Dad with Celiac) Chief Marketing Officer

Jayme (Mom) VP Operations

Blake (21)

Jacob (17 Celiac)

Keep up to date with us, the awards, and future buyer guides at GlutenFreeBuyersGuide.com

CELIAC SURVEY

We polled over 600 people with celiac disease
with the intent to make you feel not so alone.

Would you recommend
Celiac Disease screening
(blood test) for all?

63% Yes

37% No

Presented by The 2022 Gluten Free Buyers Guide

YOU'RE NOT ALONE

Notes:

Notes:

Notes:

Notes:

COMING SOON - REGISTER NOW

THE 2023
GLUTEN FREE
AWARDS HOSTED BY
THE GUIDED BUYER.COM

Printed in Great Britain
by Amazon